Pastoral Ministry In The AIDS Era:
Focus On Families And Friends
Of Persons With AIDS

Pastoral Ministry In The AIDS Era:

Focus On Families And Friends Of Persons With AIDS

Louis F. Kavar

The Care Giver Book Series
The College of Chaplains
Schaumburg, Illinois

Woodland Publishing Company, Inc.
Wayzata, Minnesota

Pastoral Ministry In The
AIDS Era:

Focus On Families And Friends
Of Persons With AIDS

BV
4460.7
.K38
1988

Copyright © 1988 Louis F. Kavar
Library of Congress Card No. 88-50082
International Standard Book No. 0-934104-07-7

MANUFACTURED IN THE
UNITED STATES OF AMERICA

Contents

Foreword 9

1. Misconceptions About AIDS 13
   We Are Powerless In The Face of AIDS 13
   AIDS And People With AIDS Are to Be Feared 14
   Medical Science Is The Only Answer To AIDS 15

2. Pastoral Ministry With Families: An Overview 19

3. The Family In Crisis 23
   The Experience Of Crisis 23
   Toward A Pastoral Assessment
   Of The Family System 24
   Family Response To Crisis 30
   The Story of Tim's Family 33

4. Living The Long Haul 37
   Transition Into The Chronic Phase of Illness 37
   The Relationship With The Intimate Partner 38
   Parenting And The Person With AIDS 45
   Supporting The Chosen Family 51
   The Role Of The Pastoral Minister In The
   Chronic Phase 55

5. Living Through Death 57

Pastoral Ministry In The AIDS Era:

Focus On Families And Friends Of Persons With AIDS

Foreword

Scarcely a day passes without hearing something about AIDS. We sip morning coffee while reading newspaper headlines reporting of AIDS. We settle back for a quiet evening at home and discover a favorite T.V. program pre-empted for a drama featuring a family in crisis because of AIDS. AIDS education appears on the agenda for P.T.A. meetings, service organization luncheons and church seminars. Dating services offer AIDS-testing for their members. Buttons, bumper stickers, billboards and T.V. spots convey various messages about AIDS. In addition to the reminders of AIDS surrounding us, an estimated ten per cent of the U.S. population has known personally someone with AIDS. While the so-called "AIDS virus," HIV (Human Immunodeficiency Virus), is transmitted through body fluids, one can indeed metaphorically say that AIDS is "in the air."

Obviously a medical response to the AIDS epidemic is essential, but it is not the only vital response. Those who struggle to live with AIDS, be they persons with AIDS themselves or family and friends close to them, all need the support and encouragement to explore the difficult, spiritual questions. Pastoral ministry here means to be present to help them explore courageously these difficult questions and to insist that no one settle for easy, pious or moralistic answers.

I have found that the experience of AIDS can be transformed from despair into possibility, from curse into blessing and from death into life. The purpose of this book is to examine how these transformations can occur in the lives of those closest to people with AIDS through the support of pastoral ministers.

At the conclusion of a recent radio talk show I was asked by the host, "What do the churches need to learn to be equipped to face the problem of AIDS?" I began my response by noting the relevance of the question. As a Christian speaking to members of my own tradiiton, I believe that to be equipped to face the problem of AIDS, we need to learn one elementary thing: to be the church of Jesus Christ. While this response is indeed simple, it has far reaching implications for the Christian community.

The mission of the church is to share the love of God with all people, at all times and in all places, no matter what the circumstances may be. God does, in fact, care for us in a personal way, and the providence of God attends to us. Serious pastoral ministry in the context of AIDS deeply challenges us to be renewed in our call to share the unconditional love of God for all people, regardless of their station in life.

In much of this book I will consider what it is simply to be a pastoral presence to those who may be different from ourselves. These considerations are rooted in the Biblical tradition, following the example of Jesus who shared God's love with tax collectors, Samaritans and undesirables, as well as the example of Paul who brought the good news to the Gentiles.

At the same time a careful reading of the text will indicate its limits regarding inclusiveness. It is bound by my own experience as a white, middle class, American male. All but one case study included here refers to a white family. All the families spoken of here are of middle and upper class backgrounds. Most of the families whose experiences have been shared have a gay or bisexual man as a member. The text does not specifically deal with other AIDS situations such as the occurrence of transfusion-induced AIDS, AIDS contracted by I.V. drug abusers through the sharing of needles, the experience of foster families of AIDS children and women who contract AIDS. Statistically, gay and bisexual men make up the largest percentage of persons with AIDS, and it is with these people and their families that the bulk of my ministry has been experienced. It is this experience which forms the basis for the considerations of this book.

I have attempted to share what I have found to be important and helpful in ministering to the families and friends of persons with AIDS. I am personally encouraged by the redemptive possibilitiy given the Church through the tragic phenomenon of this illness. While the suffering of even one person is too great a cost, the hope which AIDS brings us in the Christian community is that our vision can be broadened once again to include the lives of those who for too long have not been taken seriously, the lives of the modern *anawim,* the poor ones whom God has uniquely chosen.

Rev. Louis F. Kavar
Christmas, 1987

1. Misconceptions About AIDS

As pastoral ministers, we are bound sooner or later to enter the lives of those who have been deeply touched by AIDS. Before we do so, however, we must examine briefly some of what it means to live in a society where AIDS is metaphorically "in the air." As members of society, we are shaped and carried by the beliefs, mores and attitudes which pulsate through our culture. Within the context of AIDS, these pulsations are often laden with misunderstanding, fear and prejudice. It is from these fears and misunderstandings that several misconceptions about AIDS have grown. As people of faith it is essential to explore these misconceptions and allow redemptive light to shine through this crisis of AIDS. Consider for example, the following three misconceptions about AIDS.

Misconception #1: We are powerless in the face of AIDS.

AIDS: a fatal syndrome; a death sentence. Recently, one of my clients announced, "If I get tested and have the virus, I'll just end it all right there! Why bother to live? What's the use? They can't do anything anyway!"

Unfortunately these are not unique or unusual words; I have heard these sentiments and attitudes expressed all too often, in many ways.

AIDS. The word stares back at us. Those of us who have already been personally touched by the fate of AIDS ask desperately, "Why me?" Others among us wonder, "Will I be next? How close will it come to me?"

This time in the history of AIDS is indeed a crisis. It is now that we need to be reminded of the meaning of the Chinese symbol for the word crisis—a dangerous opportunity—and re-examine our stance before AIDS.

As a therapist, I firmly believe that crisis necessitates appropriate intervention. I also believe that the secret of effective therapy, whether it be crisis intervention or long term treatment, is to re-shape, re-structure or re-frame the perception of the event; to see it in a new way. In this crisis, we need to re-frame our image of AIDS from the ominous villain in the face of which we are powerless, to that of a truly serious illness, yet one with which people do live, from which we can learn and through which we can be empowered.

The largely unspoken reality of AIDS is that while approximately half of those diagnosed with AIDS die within 18 months, ten per cent of people with AIDS are living after five years. In addition, many people with AIDS have found that changes they have made in their lives since their diagnosis have dramatically increased the quality and level of meaningfulness of their lives. A person with AIDS, diagnosed four years ago, told me recently, "I am more alive today than I ever was before AIDS."

Misconception #2: AIDS and people with AIDS are to be feared.

It is only reasonable, given the level of potency ascribed to AIDS, that this syndrome would be so inordinately feared. For example, phrases such as "AIDS-anxiety" and "AIDS-phobia" have entered our vocabulary. Yet, the truth is that AIDS is less potent than popular thinking would have us believe. The virus which causes AIDS, HIV, is transmitted in clearly specific ways. Other viral strains are equally transmissible, as hepatitus B, or even more highly transmissible, as the case of airborne T.B. Many other diseases result in untimely, unpleasant death, as lung or bone cancer. There is something more at work with the fear of AIDS than the lack of understanding medical research, the tragedy of death at a young age or the growing rate of HIV-infection. I submit that beneath many well-grounded fears encountered in this public health crisis is the fear of people who are different from ourselves, people whom we do not understand, people against whom we have many societal prohibitions.

The statistics are clear: 65 percent of people with AIDS are gay or bisexual men; 17 percent are intravenous drug users; 25 percent are black; 14 percent latino. Of women with AIDS, 52 percent are black and 25 percent are latina. Of children with AIDS, 59 percent are black; 21 percent latino; 1 percent Asian.

These groups, various minorities in American society, confront some of the deepest fears of the majority—fears about our personal identities. AIDS forces us to look long and hard at issues of sexuality, race and culture. In addition we live in a society fixated on the appeal of youthfulness. The 1980's version of the American dream of upward mobility has become a nightmare as many of the brightest and best face death before mid-life. AIDS is indeed a cruel confrontation of the status quo.

Therefore we would do well to examine carefully our own fear about AIDS as we work with those whose lives have been engulfed by this crisis. We need to ask ourselves, "What is it that we fear? Are our fears based in our discomfort with ourselves or prejudice toward those different from ourselves? Are we afraid of seeing life differently? Of finding it not to be what we expected?"

As pastoral ministers, this examination takes a more specific focus. Our call is to proclaim God's love for all people, at all times, in all situations. How do we demonstrate a pastoral care for the people of God if we ourselves are bound by fear? Realizing that God's perfect love indeed casts out all fear—even the fear of AIDS—we need to ask, "Is my view of AIDS and the person with AIDS consistent with my theology of suffering and illness? What do I believe about AIDS? Is AIDS something to be healed . . . to be repented of? Is AIDS and opportunity for spiritual growth? What is the good news that I proclaim to those whose lives are touched by AIDS?"

I believe that only through continual examination of our fears in the face of AIDS are we enabled to be channels for the grace needed in this crisis.

Misconception #3: Medical science is the only answer to AIDS.

The most common way in which we attempt to cope with our fears and feelings of helplessness in the face of AIDS is through seeking out the most current medical knowledge and research. To develop awareness of the transmission of HIV, to determine appropriate methods of risk reduction and to identify the implications of HIV antibody testing is important. Further, it is imperative that quality research continue tracing the natural history of HIV infection as well as exploring issues of treatment and vaccine development. There can be no doubt that equipped with accurate understandings of this syndrome, the hysteria experienced in American society due to AIDS can be reduced.

Simultaneously, the quest for scientific knowledge contains an operative assumption. Too often we implicitly believe that, armed with the right bit of knowledge, everything will be all right once more. In the words of a colleague: "If they would find a vaccine, we could go back to the way things were. Life would be OK again."

We need to face the reality that the problem of AIDS will be with us for a long time. Even if a potential vaccine were found today, years would be required to complete the clinical trials which are part of drug testing. In addition, manufacturing and distributing new drugs would impose still more delays.

The challenge, then, becomes how to live with AIDS. We have begun this process on a psychological level by learning to cope with illness. But coping really is not living fully. Now we must ask the spiritual question, "What is the meaning of life in the context of AIDS?"

Those who live successfully with AIDS have found answers to these questions. The answers are so personal that they often sound prosaic, but are nonetheless real. Let us take the case of the man mentioned earlier who stated that he felt more alive after his diagnosis with AIDS.

Steve is a 34 year old gay white male who was diagnosed as having AIDS about four years ago. He has described his health during this time as a roller-coaster ride, ranging from dehydration due to diarrhea, to hope from promising new drugs, to temporary blindness due to drug toxicity.

When first diagnosed, Steve's family, who knew he was gay for several years, were in shock. They struggled between wanting to be supportive and fearing their own infection. Many of Steve's friends pulled away from him. His lover of four years left him. He truly felt abandoned.

As time went on, Steve grieved his diagnosis as did his family. But he created the opportunity to heal many wounds in his relationship with his father. Also, in time, a few of his old friends returned while Steve made new ones.

Today, Steve has found a much greater intimacy in his relationships and a new freedom in his family life. This new freedom with his father includes at least daily phone conversations as well as doing things together as they had never done before. Steve recently noticed at a family gathering that he was the only one of the sons that his father embraced. Steve found new life in the face of AIDS.

What brought the change? Steve recounts a long night walk at the beach alone. "As I watched the waves roll in and the stars in the sky," he said, "I had this strange feeling. It was like I was part of something bigger than I ever thought about before. My being sick didn't matter much right then. I realized that I was really free and could do whatever I wanted. I decided I wanted something different with my family. I wanted friends who really meant something." With the help of a minister whom Steve knew socially, he began to take steps based on this new insight. That was the beginning of his new life—a new life which the pastoral minister can help the person with AIDS to find.

2. Pastoral Ministry With Families: An Overview

Tom lays quietly in the bed of a private room on the ninth floor of University Hospital. He is staring off into space, seeming not to notice my entrance to the room. His breathing is strained as an oxygen mask hisses while resting on the pillow beside his head. The room is dark and the shades drawn. A bit of light peers around the half opened door. Less than twenty-four hours ago Tom's worst fears were confirmed. A physician informed Tom that the tests confirm that his difficulty in breathing was caused by Pneumocystis carinii pneumonia, a parasitic infection of the lungs due to AIDS.

As Tom and I speak over the next two hours, I learn about many of Tom's feelings and fears. Tom is a gay man, age 28. He and his lover have been together for four years. It has been a good relationship for Tom, yet he wonders if his lover will now leave because of the diagnosis of AIDS. Tom has heard that such things are common, even though his lover, David, has assured him of his fidelity.

I ask about Tom's parents. They are on vacation with his younger sister until the end of the week. Tom seems just as glad, more or less relieved by their absence. He had not called them to let them know about his hospitalization. Tom doesn't know how he'll share the diagnosis with them. Yes, they know he is gay. "They sort of accepted it, but they don't like it," he says. "They're nice enough to David. Mom does get him a Christmas present. But they really don't approve."

Tom explains that he really never felt that he lived up to his father's expectation. His father, Tom, Sr., is a bank executive while Tom, Jr., is a craftsman, making specialty wood furniture. "Dad and I never talked much. We just went our own separate ways."

Marie, Tom's mother, is active in many community organizations, somewhat of a professional volunteer. "Everybody loves Mom. She'll do anything for anyone. She's always smiling and happy and never forgets a name or a face."

Whether the locus of ministry is a hospital, church or other facility, most often our initial pastoral encounter is with an individual presenting a concern. From this encounter we may later become directly involved with the family system.

In the case of health care chaplaincy, we most often meet a patient and through the patient come in contact with the patient's family. This was true in ministry with Tom. (Later I shall discuss the ministry to Tom's family.) Our practical experience, and most often our pastoral training, has best equipped us to deal first with the individual and then with the family members. For these reasons pastoral care with families often provides for the needs of individual family members rather than the family system as a unique entity in need of care.

The field of family systems therapy creates a necessary option for pastoral intervention with families. From this perspective, the family system is regarded as a living entity in itself. The perceptions of individual family members point to the larger picture in which can be seen the interactions of the family system. Each family system maintains certain patterns according to which the individual members interrelate. Tracking and in turn re-shaping (re-framing) these family system patterns creates new possibilities for family interaction.

In working with families of people with AIDS, it is not sufficient simply to maintain a model for family systems. Because the family of the person with AIDS is confronted by serious illness, a model which accounts for the family system faced with chronic illness is essential.

Psychiatrist John S. Rolland, writing in *Family Process* (26:1987, pp. 203-221) proposes such a conceptual framework for viewing chronic illness and the life cycle which brings together three evolutionary dimensions: the illness itself, individual and family life cycles. From Rolland's perspective, the illness, AIDS, is described as (1) having a gradual onset which can provide more time and opportunity for adjustment for both the individual and family; (2) a progressive course in which there is generally a gradual increase in the incapacitating dimensions of the illness, (3) a usually fatal outcome.

These three aspects of the biological progression of the illness, AIDS, are in turn correlated with developmental stages of living with the illness and concomitant psychic tasks.

The first stage of the life cycle of an illness is crisis. This period of crisis is characterized by the discovery of pre-diagnostic symptoms, diagnosis and the initial adjustment to the diagnosis. During the time of crisis, the person with AIDS learns to deal with illness-related symptoms, the health care environment and treatment procedures, while simultaneously establishing working relations with the health care team. At the same time, the tasks of the family system are several. They include (1) creating a meaning for the illness that maximizes the preservation of a sense of mastery and competency in the face of the illness; (2) grieving the loss of family identity prior to diagnosis; (3) moving toward an initial acceptance of the permanent change caused by the illness while maintaining a sense of continuity with the past and the future; (4) pulling together to undergo the short term crisis while developing a flexible family structure for the next stage.

The second stage in the family life cycle of illness is known as the chronic stage. It is the time of the "long haul" of the illness. The concept of "long haul" cannot be adequately grasped by the biological progression of the illness as this progression varies considerably with AIDS. The long haul of this stage is the day to day living with the illness which may be marked by constancy, progression or episodic change. Due to the usual fatality of AIDS, this stage may be experienced as living in limbo. Family hopes to resume "normal" life might indeed be realized only through the death of their loved one. The psychic task of this period is for each family member to maintain the greatest degree of autonomy while at the same time participating in mutual dependency and care taking.

The third stage in this framework is the terminal phase. This stage is marked by pre-terminal physiological deterioration, the actual death of the family member, mourning and resolution of the loss of the family member. In the pre-terminal dimension of this stage, the inevitability of death becomes apparent and dominates family life. The time of mourning is marked by issues of separation, death, grief, resolution of mourning and the resumption of "normal" family life beyond the loss.

Later in this book we will follow Tom's family and the families of several other people with AIDS through the life cycle of living with AIDS. We will examine the experience of the family system and AIDS through the perspectives of the members and their relationships to the person with AIDS. We will consider the special pastoral needs of these families. In looking in depth at a few cases, we will move towards developing certain conclusions about ministry with families and friends of persons with AIDS in a variety of pastoral settings.

3. The Family In Crisis

The Experience Of Crisis

Crisis is a dangerous opportunity. This is the meaning given crisis by the Chinese symbol for this word. The sudden, unexpected interruption of life's normalcy that we know as crisis is fraught with various, often conflicting emotions. These emotions —threat, shock, fear, anger, hesitation, disbelief, hope—underscore the elements of danger and opportunity found in the encounter with crisis. No matter how we experience a particular crisis, no matter the degree of emotional intensity in the time of crisis, the phenomenon of crisis by nature hurls us into points of decision-making and restructuring of our lives, often in significant ways. Such is true of crisis experienced in the face of AIDS.

The crisis event may indeed vary with the experience of AIDS. For the person with HIV-infection, the event which marks the crisis may be very tangible. For example, the reception of a positive antibody test result, the discovery of a Kaposi's sarcoma lesion or an experience of personal alienation, such as a friend refraining from a usual handshake or embrace. For a loved one or friend, the discovery of another's diagnosis is often a crisis event. For others the fear that AIDS may touch their lives more closely than expected may be another such event.

The effective presence of the pastoral minister early within the time of crisis can be of significant importance. The role of the pastoral minister at this time is two fold. First, the pastoral minister provides a stable, secure presence amid the insecurity created by the crisis. Secondly, the pastoral minister assesses the skills and strengths of those in the crisis to manage this period of emotional upheaval.

Pastoral assessment includes several aspects: clarification of the crisis event (i.e., identifying what happened), exploration of the individual's connection to a faith-tradition and determining the family strengths, weaknesses and resources. This dimension of the assessment explores issues such as who is family in this situation; how has this family managed with crisis events in the past; what family resources can be utilized in this crisis; and how can these resources be best mobilized?

Toward A Pastoral Assessment Of The Family System

Each of us is bonded to others in some way which we come to identify as family. These bonds may be the result of biological relatedness, legally recognized commitment (as in the case of marriage or adoption) or other intentional commitment sometimes referred to as the family of choice. The meaning of family and the importance given to these various bonds varies and differs considerably from person to person.

The field of family therapy attempts to describe and categorize various types of family constellations. This field lists various types of families such as the family of origin, the nuclear family, an extended family, a single-parent family and a blended family. It further describes the dynamics within a family system, as in the case of an enmeshed family which is bound so closely as to have turned in on itself, stunting the growth of its members. While these constellations and descriptive categories provide the professional helper with models to employ when conceptualizing family patterns, they only serve as a partial referent to the personal relatedness which is experienced as family for any one individual.

Those of us who are white, middle or upper class, North American and Christian tend to share certain definitions of family. Our primary model for family life is that of the nuclear family. Although a great number of families with whom we work are not nuclear families but single parent or blended families, we tend to believe these other family units are somehow hurting or broken because of our assumption that family wholeness and unity in based on the model of nuclear family.

Further, the intimate bonding among many people does not

easily fit any of these definitions of family. For example, a family may be comprised of several siblings with a common mother and different fathers, who are primarily cared for by an older matriarch who may be a grandmother, aunt or a biologically unrelated person. Such a family does not fit the nuclear model, but is nevertheless often bound more closely by family values of loyalty and commitment than the typical nuclear family.

Another example is the experience of family within American gay male culture. Frequently gay men maintain nominal ties with their biological families. But the real sense of family for gay men often comes through a network of close gay male associates, known as the "family of choice." While there is no single model for these networks, many gay men often report experiencing a greater sense of commitment, acceptance and care with this gay family than within their biological family.

The pastoral minister providing care in the context of AIDS must maintain a certain awareness of the breadth of family experience shared by those most at risk to this syndrome. Because of this breadth of family experience, it is crucial for the provision of sound care that the pastoral minister carefully identify the unique family system at hand.

Assessing the family system is indeed an art. In working with any minority group, it is important to remember that the minority will address the majority on the majority's own terms. For example, I once served as chaplain in a health care facility adjacent to a black urban neighborhood. I worked with many patients and families who were black. Repeatedly, I was struck by the fact that when I, a white person, would enter a black patient's room, the spoken idiom would quickly change from black to white. Such is also true when gay or lesbian people address those who are perceived to be non-gay. In this circumstance, the gay slang known as "camp" is eliminated from the conversation.

The operative question for the pastoral minister becomes how to obtain the information needed for an accurate family assessment given what is usually a perceived difference between a minority receiving care from a member of the majority. An ac curate family assessment requires that the pastoral minister somehow share the experience of the real family of the person at hand. One may begin with a direct, open-ended question like, "Would you tell me about your family?" This question would indeed give rise to significant information. Yet, this information would be limited to how the minority person perceives the pastoral minister to be defining family. Other questions may be asked, as: "Who are the important people in your life? With whom do you most enjoy sharing special times in your life, like holidays? With whom do you feel most at home?" *These* questions, asked conversationally, will elicit information about significant relationships and how these relations function with each other. From this information, the pastoral minister begins to touch the texture of the fabric which is the complex family system of the person with AIDS.

Tracking the various components of the family system, comprised of both the biological family and the family of choice, and then considering the relative importance of these components to the person with AIDS provide a solid foundation for future pastoral intervention within the family system. The importance of this foundation should not be minimized, for future ministry will be built on it.

With this foundational framework at hand, the pastoral minister can begin to fill in needed pieces of the puzzle of living effectively with AIDS. Of great importance is learning how this system —and its constituent parts—has dealt with crisis in the past. In the family system, is there experience with chronic, debilitating or terminal illness? What was the illness? How is it similar to AIDS? How was this illness experienced by the family? How did the family live with the illness? Expect similar patterns in this present health crisis.

Ministers are familiar with the fact that tracing this history is the basic stuff in crisis intervention with families. But AIDS provides a twist. This twist is the potential lack of knowledge of or comfort with the person with AIDS' life-style. For example, in the case of a gay man with AIDS, it is important to know if the biological family is aware of his sexual orientation. This information should be obtained from the person with AIDS. If the family is aware of his sexual orientation, the pastoral minister should explore how homosexuality is viewed by the family members. A diversity of opinion and comfort may exist within the family system regarding issues of sexual orientation and sexual expression. This, combined with the value the family places on mutual acceptance within the family will be indicators of how the system will cope with a gay member with AIDS. Conversely, if the biological family does not know of the member's sexual orientation, the gay person has the right to decide when and how other family members are to be informed.

In addition, there is often a difference between the acceptance of a family member who is gay and the acceptance of a lover or the extended gay family. If this is a source of tension, it is often complicated by the legal rights of members of the biological family and the attachment to and emotional support from the gay extended family felt by the person with AIDS. In this maze, it is important that the pastoral minister work to avoid estrangemnt by either segment of the broader family system since both parts of the system are of vital importance to the person with AIDS. The pastoral minister may be able to offer creative solutions to this broader family conflict by maintaining a non-polarized role.

In the case of the I.V. drug user with AIDS, there may be tensions between the biological family and I.V. drug using friends of the person with AIDS. Biological family members may suspect drug using friends of supplying drugs to the person with AIDS. Because of this suspicion, biological family members may attempt to limit contact between the person with AIDS and the other family of choice comprised of drug using friends. On the one hand, these friends may well be the only individuals with whom the person with AIDS has shared other significant experiences. On the other, the cycle of addiction severely limits the emotional support which addicted people are capable of providing. With all these complexities, it is understandable that the I.V. drug user with AIDS may experience particular isolation and a lack of personal support.

Beyond these issues related to current addiction, attention should be paid to the biological family's history of drug and alcohol use. Several recent studies explore the impact of addiction on the family system. The pastoral minister needing to explore this issue further may refer to Sharon Wegscheider's landmark text, *Another Chance: Hope and Health for the Alcoholic Family* (Science and Behavior Books, Inc., 1981).

Families with hemophiliac members also have special concerns. While a family may have lived with this particular chronic illness for some time, the experience of AIDS re-awakens many issues which may not have been fully resolved. This hereditary disease is indeed treatable through the supplemental use of clotting factors absent in the hemophiliac's blood. The threat of AIDS has resulted in this treatment being often perceived by the hemophiliac as potentially deadly. This perception may stir feelings of unresolved guilt to the hereditary nature of the disease as well as reinforce a sense of victimization.

In addition to these special issues related to the various families with members who are presently most at-risk for HIV-infection, one issue of importance for all in the family system is the possibility of previous encounters with AIDS. While AIDS may not be an illness most biological family members have first hand experience with, hemophiliac families and gay or drug using families of choice may have known others with AIDS or fear HIV-infection for themselves. The AIDS diagnosis of a loved one may bring one's deepest fears for oneself very close to the surface.

A loved one's diagnosis of AIDS carries the impact associated with the diagnosis of any terminal illness. In addition, AIDS confronts the beliefs of other family members (and all society) about sexuality, drug use, sinfulness, human frailty and mortality. Further, this diagnosis tests the capacity for human commitment and personal acceptance while challenging these beliefs which are part of the individual's worldview.

In tracing the history of how the family system has lived with serious illness and other crises, the pastoral minister will uncover the strengths and weaknesses of this system. The discovered strengths become the first line resources to be mobilized. Mobilizing these strengths can, in turn, minimize the potency of the weaknesses.

Following is a simple case example of the facets of AIDS ministry to families and friends which have been discussed in the preceding paragraphs. A health care chaplain passing the hospital chapel hears a distressed woman crying, repeating the words, "Lord, what happended to my baby." The minister enters the chapel to find a middle-aged black woman sitting in the pew rocking, while crying her lament. The chaplain sits beside her and gently asks to speak to her. The woman, named Beatrice, begins, "I lost my baby. I don't know what happened. We gave him a Christian home and tried to do him right. But we lost him." The chaplain asks what Beatrice means by losing her baby. "He's got that disease, the homosexual disease. The doctor said my Jimmy's a homosexual and a drug addict. Lord, how'd I lose my Jimmy?" Through some further exploration, the chaplain discovers that Jimmy, age 32, has just been diagnosed with AIDS.

The chaplain begins to talk through three issues with Beatrice. First, that AIDS is a disease caused by a virus. The chaplain explains that those infected with the virus can get the disease. The purpose of this explanation is to re-focus the disease away from being a gay disease. Secondly, the chaplain uses the resource of Beatrice's love for Jimmy while shifting the focus from Jimmy being "lost" to Jimmy "being ill" needing someone to care for him. The chaplain addresses Beatrice saying, "Jimmy's not lost. He's here in the hospital. He's your son, just like he's always been. But now he needs some special care. How can we see to it that Jimmy gets the care that he needs now?" Beatrice responds, "The doctor says he's a homosexual and drug addict." The chaplain moves to a third point, re-framing sexual orientation and addiction to, "That may be true, but that means that Jimmy needs someone to care for him." At a future time, the chaplain may be able to talk through some of Beatrice's feelings about homosexuality and drug use.

In this exchange, Beatrice is given the assurance that her son is not lost, implying that she did not fail as a mother by losing her child. Further, she is allowed to use the resource of a mother's love by accepting that this is still her child. Beatrice is encouraged to care for her child as before, but not mandated to be a good mother. The chaplain allows options for Beatrice to express her care by asking, "How can we see to it that Jimmy gets the care he needs now?" All these interventions are made by reframing the concepts which are difficult for Beatrice to accept. Beatrice is given the option of seeing the situation in a new way. We assume she is comfortable with the idea of a mother taking care of a child in need, has indeed done so in the past and can be empowered to do so once again.

Earlier it was stated that the primary role of the pastoral minister is to provide a stable, secure presence in the uncertainty of crisis. In reflecting further on this role I should point out that it is through this ministry of presence, simply being with those in crisis, that the unconditional love of God is perhaps best mediated. Other pastoral agendas—to evangelize, to offer sacramental ministry or to provide theologically sound answers—should not interfere with the ministry of pastoral presence at this time. Agendas such as these often are experienced as alienating by those who have not maintained a relationship with a religious tradition. Further, if those in crisis find that the pastoral minister can be counted on to be present, the relationship will often grow to where these other forms of ministry will flow into the relationship quite naturally at a later time. The initial goal of ministry in time of crisis is to be a stable presence in the midst of emotional upheaval while maintaining an authentic openness to sharing the experience of those in crisis, in particular, the experience of being family.

Family Response To Crisis

The experience of crisis is overwhelming. The human response to being overwhelmed tends to fall into two categories, "fight or flight."

Fighting the crisis of AIDS may take several forms. Fighting may be expressed as anger directed at care-givers, other family members, the person with AIDS, society, the Church or virtually anyone or anything else. As devastating as this anger may seem, it is a sign of movement, of hope and of a certain capacity to attack the problem of AIDS.

Anger is usually able to be profitably directed. There are often many tasks to perform. The diagnosis of AIDS will mean that new medical and social systems must be explored for appropriate treatment and support. Much new information will need to be processed and comprehended. This anger can be the source of energy to be tapped for this work.

Another potential fight response may be direct mobilization. Here, family members may begin almost immediately to seek out "the best possible care." This will mean varying things for different family systems but is clearly an expression of fighting AIDS.

While fighting is indeed a hopeful sign, flight should not be viewed as unhopeful. The flight response is often complex and laden with manifold issues.

Flight is often the result of the harshness of reality breaking into one's experience of the world in a way which is incomprehensible to or incongruent with one's world view. Because of this intrusion, flight may be the safety valve which allows enough steam to dissipate from the experience to begin to see the experience more clearly.

Flight also may lead to a rigid, fixed stance that does not allow for a new perspective and results in the loss of family relationships.

This latter response poses a significant problem in working with families of people living with AIDS. Among people responding this way we find the gay lover who abandons his beloved after eight years due to fear of his own infection or guilt that he may have infected his partner; or the alcoholic father who, in denying his own addiciton, disowns his only daughter who mainlines heroin; or the mother who, with her pastor's support, rejects her gay son as sinful because she secretly believes she has failed as a parent.

In these situations, flight is often the result of fear (of self or the other) rooted in misunderstanding. Those who are fearful need support and encouragement. The pastoral minister needs to maintain a supportive posture towards these members of the family system without supporting the fear or betraying the confidence of other members. Including another colleague for a team approach to this ministry or for on-going consultation in walking this confusing path may be helpful. Perhaps, in time, the opportunity will come for the person to explore the cause of their flight. The reality is that for some people, that opportunity does not come until after the death of the family member, if at all.

Increasingly, as AIDS becomes a less rare phenomenon, fewer individuals totally reject their family members with AIDS. What happens more often is that different segments of the family system are ready to cope with the illness at different times. This is often for two reasons. First, rarely do all members of the family system learn of a diagnosis at the same time. Frequently, those members with stronger emotional attachments or in closer geographic proximity are informed of the diagnosis before others. Secondly, family members will respond differently from each other, some being ready to fight, others taking some space to distance in order to examine various issues only to return at a later time and still others experiencing longer term denial about the person's illness. Given this usual staggering of sharing information and the ability to cope with that information, the family system as a whole may experience crisis for a prolonged period. Externally, the marker for initial adjustment to the diagnosis is a certain ease with which the member of the family system learns to deal with medical and supportive systems. Internally, this adjustment is the acceptance of AIDS as part of living.

The length of time involved in making this adjustment will vary for families according to many factors ranging from the availability of AIDS-related services to the family's ability to problem-solve. It is rare that such an adjustment takes less than one month, most often taking about three months, while in other cases, somewhat longer.

The Story Of Tim's Family

While chatting with congregation members during fellowship hour following Sunday service, Rita approaches her pastor and asks to speak with her privately. After they step out of ear-shot of others, Rita informs the pastor that her brother, Tim, who lives in another part of the country was diagnosed with AIDS a few weeks ago. Tim is currently in the hospital but will be discharged in about another week. He is not well enough to live alone. Their elderly mother resides in the same city and is the only relative there. Mother is willing to take in Tim, but she is probably not well enough to take care of him due to her arthritis. Tim is an active I.V. drug user. Rita asks if the pastor could meet with her family to discuss the feasibility of inviting her brother to live with them. The pastor agrees to visit Rita's home the following evening.

Arriving at Rita's home, the pastor is greeted by her husband, Eric. Although their four children are grown and live away from home, the pastor finds two of the children, Sarah and Andrew, with Rita awaiting her arrival. Sarah is a nurse at a local hospital who is married with one child and another on the way; Andrew is a first year seminarian.

As the pastor begins to talk with the family, Rita explains that Sarah has received information on AIDS from a nursing in-service held at the place of her employment and has shared it with the family. The family seems to have a clear understanding of the disease. The dicussion begins to broaden.

Sarah: I know what the literature says. I read the studies. I know there's not supposed to be anything to fear, but. . .what if they're wrong? What if my kids would get something from Uncle Tim? I don't know what I'd do.

Andrew: I don't think we have anything to be afraid of. But there are other things to think about. Look at the kind of life Uncle Tim leads. It's no wonder he's got AIDS! Professor Jones said this is God's punishment. When you look at someone like Uncle Tim, you know it's got to be.

Eric: Now, let's look at this carefully. This is your mother's brother. Whether we like how he's lived or not, we have some responsibility for him. Your grandmother can't take care of him. How she's able to stay in her own home in her condition is miracle enough. I'm just afraid of Tim using drugs here. I don't want that kind of stuff under my roof. And you know his friends will bring it to him.

The pastor asks about Tim's friends. Rita explains that Tim visits about twice a year. The family is aware that Tim has drug contacts to keep him supplied while visiting. He has never used drugs in their home but goes elsewhere to get a fix.

The pastor notes how difficult it is to talk about these matters, and then suggests that they move back to the issues which were presented initially.

Pastor: It's understandable that given the often conflicting things we see on T.V. and read in the papers about AIDS that we'd all have some fears about this disease, just as you were saying earlier, Sarah. Maybe we could talk about those fears.

The family slowly begins to share their fears about infection, as well as fears of the stigma of AIDS.

Rita: I'm not sure our friends will want to visit if Tim's here once they find out about it and what he's got. And Eric, what about people at the office?

Pastor: Do they need to know? What I mean is that not everyone has the right to know about this. You'll probably want to tell most people that you have a sick brother here, but maybe not the total diagnosis.

Andrew: But won't the talk just start? You know, rumors and everthing? How's that going to look for me at the seminary?

Pastor: Yes, there will be some people who will wonder and maybe even try to start rumors. You may lose some friends, too. That will be unfair and unfortunate. The only thing I can promise is that you have my support. I'm also sure that many people at the church will be there for you, too—if you want them to be. We've been doing some things on AIDS as part of the Christian Education Program with a lot of positive response. The AIDS program our denomination is doing in this District has also been well received. And our bishop did personally initiate that program, Andrew.

Eric: Well, we have each other. And those who won't deal with this, maybe they're really not such good friends after all.

The pastor continues to be supportive, helping the family to look at the reality of their fears of this disease and their possible rejection by friends and colleagues.

Pastor: I can see that Tim's possible use of drugs in the house may also be a concern for you.

Eric: Well, I just can't allow that in my house. (To Rita) Honey, am I wrong to say that?

Rita: No. I agree. I don't like it either.

Eric: It's illegal and it's dangerous. What if something happened?

Pastor: Those are legitimate concerns. There are drug rehab programs here willing to work with people with AIDS.

Rita: Tim won't do that. We've talked about it before.

Pastor: You may want to talk about it again. Maybe his diagnosis will be what it takes to get him to do something. But if not, you may need to set some rules for Tim. Could you do that?

Eric: Like if he uses drugs, he's out?

Pastor: That's a possibility. How would you feel about that, Rita?

Rita: I agree. But where would he go?

Pastor: That's a problem. There are no homes here for people with AIDS.

Rita: From what mom said, his friends smuggled drugs into the hospital. They shot them into his I.V. line.

Sarah: I've seen that happen.
Rita: If we don't take him, mom will. She won't say no even
            though it's too much for her.

Understanding the dilemma, the pastor tries to look for further options. Rita is planning to visit her mother later in the week. Perhaps Rita can meet with her mother and a social worker from the hospital or AIDS task force to assess realistically the situation. Perhaps Rita's mother can be given the support she needs to set appropriate limits for herself. Perhaps some other AIDS-related service provides housing in that city. When Tim is healthy enough, Rita can present him with the reality of the situation, stressing that the family wants to support him, but not his addiction. The pastor may try to make contact with the pastoral minister who can offer Rita support while visiting her mother and Tim. Clearly, all of the issues cannot be resolved completely in this visit without some further information. The pastor can provide a sense of what support is available to them if Tim moves in with Rita and Eric as well as help them set the conditions for that move.

In this situation the minister obtained a sense of the family network and provided a supportive presence while attempting to move toward creative solutions. Solutions to the complex problems of AIDS are not easy. In these entangled situations, the assurance that the family will not have to struggle alone is of great value.

4. Living The Long Haul

Transition Into The Chronic Phase Of Illness

As the family of the person with AIDS moves towards initial acceptance of the disease, the family system moves away from the closer bonding associated with the crisis period and returns to the more flexible bonding experienced prior to the crisis. This movement is associated with a return of certain feelings of normalcy about life as was known before the time of crisis. During the crisis phase, various aspects of the personal lives of family members necessarily took on a secondary importance in light of the crisis event. Those things put aside for the sake of the crisis are now able to be re-addressed, albeit sometimes in new ways. There is now movement toward the day to day living with AIDS known developmentally as the chronic phase of illness.

The experience of day-to-day living with this illness will vary from family to family. Most often there are substantial periods of constancy, when life takes on a routine quality. Familiar parts of life, as work, school and other activities, are blended with new things, like support group meetings and wellness workshops. This combination of the familiar and the new form the basis for day to day rhythms of living with AIDS.

Through these times of constancy, a gradual progression of the disease may also occur. This slow progression often takes place with the cancers associated with AIDS. In addition, normal aches and pains are often accompanied with fear and apprehension of further disease. This fear may be of a sudden, episodic illness which frequently interrupts periods of constancy, such as the infection of Pneumocystis carinii pneumonia. All these experiences form the core of the long haul associated with the chronic phase of AIDS.

During this phase, as the dust settles from the earlier crisis, many of the complex personal issues of AIDS are addressed by the family members of the person with AIDS. In this chapter we will examine some of those issues as they pertain to spouses, partners, lovers, parents and other chosen family members of people living with AIDS.

The Relationship With The Intimate Partner

With the primary mode of transmission for HIV being sexual, the intimate partner or spouse of the person living with AIDS may be the family member most deeply threatened by the diagnosis. This may take many forms. It may be wife or husband, same-sexed lover or unmarried sexual partner with whom the person with AIDS may cohabit. While these coupled relationships have similar dynamics and concerns among them, each maintains its own uniqueness.

Among the common concerns, two are perhaps most central. The first concern is whether the partner has become infected by the person with AIDS. This is surely difficult because the illness forces the loved one to face his or her own mortality.

While it may be advisable for the pastoral minister to support the partner in seeking appropriate medical treatment, including HIV-antibody testing, the pastoral minister should also help the concerned partner evaluate the quality of the treatment available. In the case of antibody testing, testing should always be preceded and followed by thorough counseling. Such pre-test counseling should include a complete history of the partner's sexual activity, sexual relations between the couple and other high risk behavior as I.V. drug usage. Such a history will assist in determining the likelihood of the partner's infection, serving as groundwork for risk reduction education, as well as clarifying what may be realistic concerns by the partner about the source of infection for the loved one.

In addition to this historical information, the partner should be educated before testing to clarify the meaning of antibody test results. The partner should be given the assurance that a positive antibody test result does not mean that the partner will later develop symptoms of the disease. This education should also be repeated after testing along with clear instructions as to principles for risk reduction, including safer-sex guidelines.

Further, both pre- and post-test counseling should allow the partner to express anger regarding the potential infection through sexual relations with the loved one. This anger is often difficult to express. The partner frequently experiences guilt over notions of what it is to be a "good wife" or "good lover." For instance, the partner may feel that to be truly loving, she or he should *not* be angry. Or perhaps because the loved one is in need of care, anger is inconsistent with providing that care. The partner may wonder, "How can I be angry when he/she is sick and could die?" The pastoral minister may serve a vital role in allowing such anger to be expressed privately, supporting its expression, while assuring the partner that feeling anger does not minimize the real care in the relationship. From this support, the partner may learn to express constructively the anger with the loved one or use its energy in coping with the illness.

Regarding issues of safer sex the partner will doubtlessly have many feelings and fears regarding future sexual relations. Because sex is often a difficult subject to discuss, the pastoral minister should encourage dialogue around these feelings. That encouragement may be for discussion of these issues with the pastoral minister, if that minister is properly informed regarding sexual issues; or may take the form of referring the partner to an appropriate professional who can address safer sex in an understanding and competent way.

Learning new ways of relating sexually is often difficult, awkward or embarassing for many people. Simply reading through a list of safer sex recommendations often does little to allay the awkwardness. Talking through the fear, as well as role-playing conversations about initiating sexual encounters can be helpful. It is important to remember that partners are often caught between the fear of their own infection and the desire to be loving, accepting and supportive of their loved one with AIDS.

The other side of the partner's fear of having been infected by the loved one is the fear that the partner may have infected the loved one, causing the disease. In this case, the partner may experience embarassment, guilt, anger and depression. Once again, it is important for the partner to express these emotions in an appropriate way and for the pastoral minister to facilitate and encourage appropriate expression.

The second common concern shared among the various forms of spousal relationships is the anxiety experienced in regard to what may be the unknown behavior of the loved one. In the case of sexual transmission of HIV, it is not unusual that the spouse is not aware that the loved one was involved in sexual activity outside the relationship. This causes a variety of difficulties, especially in the case of a wife who may not be aware of her husband's activities. A woman whose husband is secretly involved in extramarital affairs usually experiences hurt and anger when being informed of these affairs. In addition, she may experience a sense of self-doubt, wondering what she could have done to cause him to move beyond the relationship, feeling somehow responsible for his actions. In the case of a bisexual husband who is involved with another man, these feelings are further intensified for the wife, including a clear sense of betrayal. The story of Barb and Carl typify this experience.

Barb and Carl had been married for 14 years. Carl, a consultant, traveled on business regularly. Barb, with their three children, was active in parent, civic and church groups in the upper-middle class community where the family lived. Barb was a generous, gracious and accepting woman. She was readily available to meet the needs of others in a rather unassuming way.

Carl had been traveling a bit more than usual over a several month period. Feeling run down and noticably fatigued, he saw the family physician at Barb's insistence. The physician recommended further consultation which resulted in Carl's hospitalization for tests. While hospitalized, Carl, who had increasing difficulty in breathing, became suddenly ill. The tests revealed Pneumocysitis carinii pneumonia, qualifying Carl for a diagnosis of AIDS.

Over the next few weeks, Barb dutifully cared for her husband and children. She feared the loss of Carl while trying to provide a stable home life for her children. Carl returned home while continuing to convalesce.

During this time, Barb scheduled an appointment with a physician to determine if she had been infected with HIV. In discussion with the doctor, Barb stated that she and Carl did not have intercourse often and that, when they did, they used condoms and foam as a birth control device. Barb's antibody test result was negative.

Based on discussion with the physician, Barb began to wonder how Carl could have been infected with the virus. Was it some strange accident? She rarely initiated sex with Carl. Was he frustrated with her, she wondered. Could he have slept with another woman, possibly a prostitute, while away on business? It was difficult for Barb to imagine because she believed that they had a good marriage. Then Barb thought that Carl was surely lonely, being on the road so much, and that he must have just made a little mistake for which he is indeed suffering.

While Barb continued to wonder about what Carl had done, she was also glad that he seemed to be feeling better. Carl had a lot of support from several business associates, which pleased Barb, especially in light of stories she had heard about friends abandoning people with AIDS. One man in particular, a colleague with whom Carl had worked on a project in another city, called regularly. Barb had spoken to him on occasion before Carl's illness. At that time, his calls gave Barb a sense of security that if anything ever happened to Carl while away, he had friends he could count on. Now her belief that these were caring friends was reinforced.

Continuing to wonder how Carl had been infected, Barb made an appointment with her minister to talk about her concerns. Barb shared with the minister that she believed that Carl probably had sex with a prostitute while away on business. Yet, Barb was not sure. She also spoke of her hesitation in asking Carl about any of these matters because she was anxious about how Carl might respond as well as about what else she might hear. In addition, Barb felt a certain ambivalence. She was not sure that knowing really mattered at this point. What good would the information do?

The minister observed that Barb was obviously bothered by not knowing how Carl had been infected. He suggested that to put it to rest once and for all she simply ask.

The following Saturday, while their children were out for the afternoon, Barb asked Carl if she could talk with him. She explained that she didn't want to upset him, assured him that she would accept whatever he would say and asked that he honestly explain how he could have gotten AIDS. She asked if he had an affair.

Carl was shaken. He spoke slowly and deliberately. He said that he did have an affair of sorts. Barb asked what he meant. Finally, Carl blurted out that he was gay and that the man who called frequently from out of town was actually his lover.

Barb was dumbfounded. She had never expected anything like this. She did not know what to think or say. Carl tried to explain that he did love her and never wanted to hurt her. Yet, he was gay. He thought if he got married he would get over his feelings about men. But it had not worked out that way. Carl kept repeating his love for Barb.

A few days later, Barb made an appointment at a pastoral counseling center sponsored by the churches in her area. She explained her dilemma to the therapist. Barb felt angry, used and betrayed. She also wondered what was wrong with her. What could she have done to be so displeasing to Carl to want a man instead of her?

Weeks passed. When Carl was out of town on business, Barb would wonder what he was doing. During one trip, she moved her personal belongings into the guest room, deciding it was best not to share a bedroom with Carl.

Carl tried to talk with Barb about what had happened. It was too painful for her. As time went on and Carl once again became ill, suffering various effects of several different infections, Barb tried to push her personal feelings away to care for Carl.

A few weeks before his death, Carl asked if he could invite his lover, Stan, to visit for a few days. Barb agreed on the condition that Stan stay in a hotel. Carl said that he could understand Barb's wanting that and agreed that such was appropriate.

It was difficult for Barb to meet Stan. The first visit was very awkward as Barb felt this was the person to whom she lost her husband. Stan arrived with flowers for Barb, which took her by surprise. Stan was warm, friendly, and charming. Before ending his visit, he asked Barb to join him for dinner. Being too embarassed to say no, she accepted. During dinner, Stan apologized to Barb for any heartache which he might have caused her. He tried to explain his love for Carl as well as the awkwardness he felt as the third person. Barb admitted her desire to try to compete with Stan to have the final assurance of Carl's love and affection. Stan tried to explain that there was no need to compete. He went on to say that his relationship with Carl was very different than Barb's. Stan reminded Barb that Carl fathered her children, tried to provide a good home life for both Barb and the children and always returned home to her. Stan recounted many times when he felt disgruntled because Carl spoke so lovingly about Barb and the kids, knowing that he would never have that kind of relationship with Carl.

Barb repeatedly talked about this conversation with her pastoral counselor. It became a turning point for her. She gradually began to feel less responsible for Carl's actions and to understand what the counselor told her about sexual orientation. While she still felt betrayed, she began to admit feeling a certain affection for Stan. Through the support of the pastoral counselor, Barb was able to accept that she had been a good, loving wife and mother while also learning to be more self-caring and assertive.

In addition to the particular issues related to women who are married to gay or bisexual men, heterosexually married couples with a partner with AIDS experience a particular loss. Due to the perinatal transmission of HIV, future attempts at pregnancy are often unwise. Given this reality, young couples may be faced with mourning the loss of plans for future children. In addition, the possibility that young children in the biological family may have been infected with HIV may need to be explored. The recommendations made earlier regarding testing should be adapted and followed according to the age of the children.

Unmarried couples present their own unique needs. Because of the lack of legally recognized commitment, the partner in this situation may be uncertain of what role to play in the relationship. This internal confusion related to the unmarried partner's role may be magnified by the view of this relationship held by other family members. Frequently, other family members will either assume many of the care-taking duties for the person with AIDS or, in more stressful situations, simply attempt to prevent this partner from having access to the situation. Such can be true for both non-married heterosexual couples or same-sexed couples.

There are many further considerations for gay male couples where one member has AIDS. Both members of the couple are of course considered at risk for infection, but with the above stated concerns of how infection entered the relationship, two beliefs impinge heavily on gay male couples.

The first of these beliefs is actually one held in many segments of American society. The belief is that happiness will accompany the development of a coupled relationship. This belief is intensified in the gay male community, and takes on great power.

The belief may be expressed something like this: "If I find the right lover with whom I can really be myself, who will accept me unconditionally, then it won't matter if my family won't accept my being gay; it won't matter that I could lose my job and home if someone finds out that I'm gay; it won't matter what the Church has to say about my sexual orientation. I'll have a lover who will be with me and that's all that matters." While this statement is indeed an exaggeration to clarify how this belief is lived out, it does convey the sense of urgency many gay men experience in their pursuit of coupled relationships. The power of this belief among gay men is related to the experience of being a sexual minority. This experience is often marked by feelings of personal alienation and marginalization as well as other complex issues related to self-esteem. Feelings of alienation frequently lead to heightened needs for intimacy and acceptance which is especially sought in the couple relationship.

When AIDS enters the relationship, the false security provided by the relationship is yanked away. Not only is the partner faced with the illness of his beloved and his own vulnerability to the disease, but he re-confronts the vulnerability of being a gay man.

Another belief which carries a profound impact on gay male couples reads something like this: gay relationships don't last. This belief tends to be self-fulfilling. The truth of our culture is that few coupled relationships endure for life. In addition, given the inordinate needs gay coupled relations are expected to meet (based on the first belief) and the lack of societal support for these relationships, it is not surprising that maintaining such relationships is difficult.

Then AIDS enters the relationship. Many gay partners experience AIDS as the ultimate frustration of the relationship. After clearing hurdle after hurdle to make the relationship work, there is the feeling that, in the end, the myth is true: this relationship won't last. Only, now it will not last because of AIDS and there is nothing to be done about that.

In looking at the unique experience of spousal relationships and people with AIDS, the pastoral minister is again faced with the highly individualistic character of the definition of what it is to be a spouse as well as the wide variety of stresses on these relationships. The pastoral minister can be present to share in the process of sifting through the diverse needs and feelings of partners who have been confronted and burdened by the diagnosis of AIDS.

Parenting And The Person With AIDS

The discovery of a child's AIDS diagnosis is a traumatic event for virtually every parent. Regardless of the age of the child, parents of a child with AIDS are confronted with the untimeliness of a usually terminal disease. Having a child with such a diagnosis is often experienced as something both unreal and unnatural. Parents experience a high degree of frustration, perhaps best expressed by the phrase, "This isn't the way life is supposed to be." It is the usual expectation that parents will grow old and die, being buried by their children. The reality of AIDS subverts this seemingly usual progression. Instead, middle-aged parents often provide care for their child during various stages of this disease while potentially moving to face the death of the child.

In addition to the trauma related to the reordering of life and death due to this usually terminal disease, parents often experience a sense of failure in fulfilling their parental role. A common cultural belief concerning parenting purports that good parents raise their children in such a way as to insure the child's success in life. Conversely, a lack of success in a child's life, however that be measured, must be the result of some parental failure. Clearly, this belief has severe shortcomings and places an inordinate degree of responsibility for a child's adult life with the parents.

Yet, because of this belief, the diagnosis of AIDS presents parents with a sense of failure on two counts. The first is the potential death of a child. Death can indeed be construed as a lack of success in life; in fact, as the ultimate failure. The belief of parental responsibility places the failure of death at the parent's doorstep. In some bizarre way, it may be inferred from this view that the parents must not have adequately taught the child survival skills. Secondly, the very diagnosis of AIDS points to some parental failure when considering the diagnosis from the viewpoint of belief. That a person is diagnosed with AIDS is often interpreted as that person having done something wrong. The wrongdoing, as it is labeled here, may be homosexuality, drug use or sexual activity outside of marriage. This experience of parental failure is intensified in the case of hereditary hemophilia, in which a mother often feels responsible for her child's illness, or in the case of perinatal transmission of HIV.

These issues are particularly nuanced when included with the cycle of poverty which is often too much a part of the lives of people of color and I.V. drug users with AIDS. In many cases, the parental goal amidst poverty is to teach survival. Just making it, day-to-day, is the core of poverty living. The death of a child, for any reason, be it infant mortality, accident, or AIDS, is a reminder of the harshness of life and the need to teach survival. Beyond this survival issue, families living in poverty must face the inequities of our health care systems and the family's own inability to provide their loved one with more adequate health care. Given these complex issues, families of poverty who live with AIDS are rarely as concerned with issues of drug use or sexual orientation and activity as they are with survival needs and trying to maintain family unity by taking care of each other to the best of their ability.

For families of the majority, parents are faced with the issue that their children may not have turned out to be who they were hoped to be. This is indeed the case for parents who did not know their child was gay, a drug user or sexually active. This new reality forces parents to deal simultaneously with the diagnosis of the child while adjusting to new or perhaps not fully understood information about their child's life.

A helpful booklet has been published by the Philadelphia chapter of Parents and Friends of Lesbians and Gays (P.O. Box 15711, Philadelphia, PA 19103). It is titled "Coming Out To Your Parents," and describes six stages of understanding which parents often go through in learning to accept a lesbian or gay child. These stages are applicable for parents confronted with *any* new or uncomfortable information which they may learn about their children. These stages include shock, denial, guilt, expression of feeling, decision-making and acceptance.

The stage of shock is part of the experience of crisis described in the preceding chapter. Shock is a certain numbness which permits the new information to be kept at bay for a short time. Shock is a response to news which is so distressing that it needs to be avoided before it can be heard.

As this news begins to be heard, shock gives way to denial. Denial serves the important function of shielding the individual from what may be unpleasant beliefs about the thing which is being denied. In this situation, the basic denial response is that the news simply cannot be true.

When denial has fallen away, guilt may result. The experience of guilt is related to the belief that the parents are somehow responsible for their child's behavior or lifestyle. Parents may wonder what they have done to cause their child's homosexuality, drug use or other behavior. As parents relinquish control over their child, accepting that they have not caused this aspect of the child's life, parents in turn learn to relate with the child on a more adult-to-adult level. This allows parents to express feelings— anger, hurt, disappointment, frustration, sadness—which they may experience due to their child's lifestyle or behavior.

Once these varied emotions can be expressed and worked through, parents are in a place to decide how they will live with this news about their child. This decision-making process leads to some form of acceptance of the child for whom the child truly is.

In the crisis phase of the illness, parents, in effect, move through these stages in learning to live with AIDS. The completion of that stage is moving to an initial acceptance of the disease. In the chronic phase, parents work through these stages in relation to their child's lifestyle. As stated earlier, it is not unusual that a parent may not have known about a child's sexual activity, orientation or drug use prior to the diagnosis. These parents are faced with the heavy burden of moving through these complex stages on two levels. Other parents may have known about their child's lfiestyle, but may not have explored their own feelings of guilt or other emotional responses to this information in order to reach a level of acceptance with which they can live. Such is true of Tom and Marie, the parents of Tom, Jr., introduced earlier in this book.

Tom and Marie had known that Tom, Jr. was gay for several years. While they were not suprised when he came out to them, it was news that was very difficult for them to hear. Since the first discussion, neither Tom nor Marie spoke about his sexual orientation with Tom, Jr., but they did speak of it between themselves.

Both Tom and Marie felt responsible for Tom, Jr. being gay. He was born at a time when Tom was starting to climb the corporate ladder, working longer hours while not spending as much time as he would with their other son, Bill. Marie tried to assume many parental responsibilities in Tom, Sr.'s absence. Marie believed that she had probably been too dominating in Tom, Jr.'s life.

Marie also worried that she had driven Tom, Jr. away from the family. They both remembered him as strongly exerting his independence when finishing high school and continuing through college. Tom, Sr. did not know how to deal with his son, but loved him greatly, trying to support Tom, Jr. by providing him with the best education available and, later, helping him to establish his first wood-working shop. He was proud of Tom, Jr.'s work and regularly pointed out to his colleagues a certain chair in his office which Tom, Jr. had made. But Tom, Sr. never knew how to tell his son how proud he was and how much he loved him.

Tom and Marie met regularly with their pastor for support since Tom, Jr.'s diagnosis of AIDS. During that time, the pastor explained some of the complexities of sexual orientation and the various theories of its causes. The pastor attempted to help them see that this, their son, was a grown adult, almost 30 years of age. He was indeed capable of and responsible for his own decisions.

Several months after Tom, Jr. had been diagnosed with AIDS, when he was back to work and doing quite well, the pastor suggested a meeting the Tom, Marie, and Tom, Jr. to discuss how they felt about Tom's being gay and having AIDS. Marie said that she would not want to say anything to her son that would hurt him as he has had enough pain to deal with. The pastor, responding empathically, emphasized that as an adult, Tom, Jr. needed to learn to cope with his parents' feelings. Marie then wondered if the stress of such a discussion would be good for Tom, Jr. as stress weakens the immune system. The pastor pointed out that Tom, Jr. was doing well and that surely his counselor and AIDS support group could help him deal with any stress from this simple meeting. The pastor added that he would be present to be sure that this conversation between adults did not become too stressful for Tom, Jr.

Listening to this discussion, Tom, Sr. asked the pastor if he really thought that talking would help, bottom line, that is. The pastor stated the belief that talking would help. As Tom, Sr. put it, "Given that we've nothing to lose, let's do it."

The following week, the pastor met with Tom, Marie and Tom, Jr. for about two hours. Tom, Jr. began somewhat angrily, stating that he had not experienced the love of his father and that Marie simply did things for the sake of appearance. Tom, Sr. responded first, explaining that he never really understood his son, but loved him greatly. He recounted the many things that Tom, Jr. had done to make him proud. Marie, crying, explained how she had caused her son so much pain by making him gay and that it was because of her that he now had AIDS. Tom explained that no one caused his sexual orientation and that he simply was who he was. He stated he was comfortable being gay, despite the pressure of society, which was a problem, but one with which he could live. Tom, Jr. reminded his mother that no one causes AIDS, but that a virus does. He further stated that he only wanted their love and understanding.

Marie and Tom, Sr. explained that their son indeed had their love even though they really didn't understand a lot about his life. They recounted times they felt their love had been thwarted and that they had been hurt by his actions.

The discussion continued through more tears and anger as they heard each other's statements of love, hurt, and confusion. Before ending, the family members were holding and comforting each other. Each left with new insight into the other.

This was not the last discussion that occurred surrounding some of the issues raised during this meeting, but it was the most intense and emotional. During the following weeks, Tom, Jr. began to spend more time with his parents, even meeting his father at work for lunch. Tom and Marie asked to meet with some of Tom and his lover, David's, friends. As it turned out, this discussion, convened by the pastor, was a turning-point in healing this relationship between parents and their son, opening communication that had been closed too long. The power of this relationship became a certain new life in the midst of AIDS.

Supporting The Chosen Family

In terms of pastoral care, perhaps the most neglected segment of the family system is what may be called the "chosen family" of the person with AIDS. The chosen family is comprised of those non-biologically related intimate companions of the person with AIDS toward whom that person regularly looks for emotional support and care. The type of bonding existing among these individuals has a quality more similar to that which is associated with families than that of friends.

In the context of AIDS, chosen families are most common among gay men, but may also exist among drug users with AIDS.

Because chosen families lack the more formal bonds of biological families and because the lives of chosen family members may not be readily apprehended by the pastoral minister, such families often do not receive the pastoral support which may be helpful for them during the time of illness. Beyond this, biologicial family members may attempt to exclude the chosen family members on the basis that they are not "real family" or because they are perceived as the source of their loved one's illness. In addition, chosen family members may be a reminder to biological family members of their loved one's lifestyle, which the biological family may prefer to forget or reject.

Chosen family members often play a vital role in relation to the person with AIDS. These family members have usually been the most intimate people in the recent life of that person. These may be the only people who can relate to or accept the lifestyle of the person with AIDS. Because of their privileged position in relation to the person, these members often are able to provide significant support.

In addition to their support of the person with AIDS, chosen family members can be a source of support to the biological family. Chosen family members can help educate the biological family about issues related to the person's lifestyle. In addition, these friends may often assist in tangible care-taking of the person with

AIDS, a support which may, in turn, be a relief to the biological family.

Chosen family members often have their own particular needs. Members of this segment of the family system are often also at risk for HIV infection. Some members may already be infected or experience various forms of illness due to infection. Many chosen family members have already known of other people with AIDS, some of whom may have lost a substantial number of friends to this disease. This segment of the family may be all too familiar with the horror of AIDS and fear that they too may one day be a fatality to this syndrome. Because of this fear, chosen family members may experience periods marked by a clear denial of AIDS itself or denial of death from this disease. Once again, the pastoral minister should remember that denial is an important coping strategy which is itself a survival mechanism.

The following conversation illustrates some of the experience of gay men confronted by the diagnosis of a close friend with AIDS.

Kevin: I visited Greg at the hospital today.

Dan: How's he doing?

Kevin: Not too badly, all things considered.

Dan: That's good, I guess. Y'know, this is his third trip in and I haven't been able to get myself to visit this time.

Kevin: That's not like you. You're normally the one telling me how he's doing. What's your problem?

Dan: I don't know. It's just hard for me this time.

Kevin: What do you mean? It's not like you've never seen anyone with AIDS before! You know you're not going to get that stuff by visiting.

Dan: Yeh, I know. It's just different this time. I don't know what it is. (pause) Greg makes the ninth friend of mine to get it! Damn disease!

Kevin: What's wrong, Dan?

Dan: Why Greg? After all he's been through. And on top of it, after all the things he does for everybody. He's the best friend anyone could want. What did he ever do to deserve this?

Kevin: He's done the same things you and I have. You know that.

Dan: Listen. I know Greg's been safe. He's been safer than me. But we know about that stuff now. I didn't know what this kind of safe was before, like when I was with Tom. That was back in 1982. Do you know what all I let him do to me? Then I found out he was running around like some cheap whore! I dumped him fast. Do you know what he could have given me? I didn't do anything different than anyone else. And neither did Greg!

Kevin: I hear you. But I know that I'm okay. It was such a relief when I got tested. And I'm going to make sure I don't get it!

Dan: I know what you mean. Do you know how I found out I was okay? We had physicals at work. They tested me and I didn't even know it. The nurse read off this list of test results and she comes out with "HIV antibody—negative." I almost fell off the chair! How can they test you without telling you?

Kevin: Yeh, they're doing it, alright.

Dan: And what if I would have been positive. Would she have just read off, "HIV antibody—positive" and gone on to the next one?

Kevin: I hear you. It's not right at all! But they don't care if we get it and die. They just want to test to know who to stay away from.

Dan: I guess so. But what's to say we won't get it?

Kevin: I'm not going to get AIDS!

Dan: But what if a rubber breaks and you get it?

Kevin: I'm not into anal sex. And I'm careful about who I do it with!

Dan: What if you meet someone and things are going well and you fall in love. You know you're a sucker for falling in love. Then, before you go to bed for the first time, you find out he's positive. What would you do?

Kevin:	Safe sex. It works.
Dan:	Would you kiss him? What if you already kissed, you know, really kissed? Would you let him do it again?
Kevin:	Stop doing this to me! I don't know.
Dan:	Does it scare you like it scares me?
Kevin:	I was out of town on that business trip a couple weeks ago. I met this really nice guy. We were talking for a long time and I really like him. He was bright and warm and seemed to have his act together. I felt like I could really like this guy and be really at-home with him. Then he told me he had ARC.
Dan:	Well, what happened?
Kevin:	I hope he couldn't tell, but I was stunned. "Why him?" I asked myself. He was really someone I wanted to get to know.
Dan:	Did you get his phone number?
Kevin:	No. He lives out of town.
Dan:	But you always said you'd move for the right guy.
Kevin:	No. It hurt too much. I got back to my hotel room and cried like a baby.
Dan:	I do that a lot, too.
Kevin:	Well...what about Greg? He was asking about you. Do you want to visit him together?
Dan:	Yeh, that would help a lot.
Kevin:	I'll tell jokes and keep everybody laughing.
Dan:	That's what you do best! How about after work tomorrow?

Because of the distance between many gay men and traditional religion, it may be difficult for most gay men to share these feelings with a pastoral minister. This is also related to issues addressed in the preceding chapter regarding how minority groups speak to those they perceive to be part of the majority. It is for this reason that a case example of a frank conversation between two gay men has been used to illustrate their experience.

The pastoral minister may best approach gay members of the chosen family with the assumption that the experience of a companion with AIDS carries with it assorted feelings, including fears for oneself, anger regarding the injustice of AIDS and relational distress. The pastoral minister may begin by offering support by speaking to these chosen family members in the absence of the person with AIDS, asking if they have known of others with HIV-infection or how they are doing in the present situation. Even if deeper conversation does not ensue, heart-felt support will be sensed, being a source of strength both at that time and in the future.

The Role Of The Pastoral Minister In The Chronic Phase

Throughout the chronic phase of illness, family members most often explore their relationships with each other and the person with AIDS. Old differences and hurts re-surface. New information regarding the AIDS diagnosis and lifestyle issues come to the foreground. While the various members of the family experience this information in different ways, all members go through a process of sifting and sorting this information in an attempt to make sense of this confusing life experience.

Throughout this time, the pastoral minister can serve as a support and facilitator of this process, clarifying the experience, creating and supporting avenues of openness needed to allow healing to occur among family members.

Through this process of healing family relationships the family moves to find life and meaning in the context of AIDS.

5. Living Through Death

The grim reality is that of those diagnosed with AIDS in the United States between January, 1981, and June, 1987, 58 percent had died by June 22, 1987. These statistics from the Centers of Disease Control, (AIDS Weekly Surveillance Report of June 22, 1987) confirm our fears of the usually terminal outcome of AIDS.

Lest we be without hope, this same report notes that nine percent of those diagnosed in 1981, were living in June of 1987. This percentage will surely increase as new treatments are tested and found effective.

Yet, for most people with AIDS, death will come within five years. People with AIDS will live varying periods of time, some not surviving their first case of Pneumocystis carinii pneumonia, while others will live for six or seven years. This difference should not be taken lightly as it will have a profound effect not only for the person with AIDS and the family system, but also on how care for the family is provided. Care based on the assumption of a quick death fails to support the day-to-day concerns of living with AIDS while removing hope for life with this syndrome.

The third developmental phase of living with AIDS, the terminal stage, may be marked by the inevitability of death which becomes apparent, dominating the life of the family system. The reality of death is most clear when the person with AIDS suffers from the slow progression of cancer or the wasting syndrome which is associated with AIDS. There may be assorted forms of debilitation and disfigurement, including the loss of psycho-motor functioning, seizure disorders and other deficits associated with AIDS dementia complex.

As with other forms of seriously debilitating terminal illness, family members are often caught between internal conflicts of not wanting to lose their loved one and wishing that the ordeal would soon be over, all the while experiencing significant distress at the suffering of their loved one.

For other people with AIDS, death may come more suddenly especially as a result of an AIDS-related infection. In such a situation, family members may be less resolved in their feelings about the death of their loved one due to the more sudden form of death.

Lastly, the death of the person with AIDS may come at any point of the illness through suicide. The phenomenon of AIDS-related suicide has not been studied extensively. Anecdotally, such attempts seem to occur more frequently with AIDS than with other terminal illnesses.

The reason for such suicides and suicide attempts are varied, but may include the multiple loss of friends to AIDS, fear of AIDS-related discrimination, unsettled issues of personal identity, lack of social or financial support, fear of family rejection or the desire not to be a burden or stigma for loved ones.

Once again, anecdotally, it seems that while family members still experience issues of survivors' guilt related to the suicide of the person with AIDS, these family members may have had a clearer suspicion of the person's suicidal ideation than is the case in other situations. This, in addition to certain potential feelings of relief that the person with AIDS has died, complicates issues of survivors' guilt. These are clearly issues in need of further study.

The family's ability to move through the experience of the death of a loved one with AIDS is very much dependent on the family's ability to sift through the issues outlined in the preceding chapter on the chronic phase of illness. For families who have resolved the variety of issues related to lifestyle or the disease itself, the dying process can be a rich experience, a "happy death" as it has been called in some Christian traditions. This resolution does not mean that all family members have positive, affirming views toward their loved one's lifestyle, but instead have made peace with the reality of the situation.

For those families who have not experienced such a resolution (unfortunately, that is the case for most families) the dying and death of the loved one intensifies this lack of resolution, increasing the sense of tension and discord among family members. Such is the case with Albert and Gary, and Albert's mother, Louise.

Albert, a gay man in his early 30's, lived with his lover of several years in an urban area. Albert was raised in the country outside this city, where his parents continue to maintain a farm.

Throughout the early part of his illness, Louise rarely had contact with her son. Albert called regularly, but Louise kept conversations brief. Albert was told that he could visit but only if he visited without his lover, Gary. Albert was resentful that the spouses of his sisters and brothers were welcome in the family home while Gary was not, and so he did not visit. Instead, he regularly invited his parents to his home for dinner—invitations which were also declined.

As Albert became more ill, he decided not to return to the hospital but to follow a home hospice progam with the support of several gay friends. When Louise realized how much her son's health had deteriorated, she began to make weekly visits to her son's apartment. She always brought with her several bags of groceries but never entered the apartment. Finally, on the day Albert was dying, Louise happened to visit while Albert's friends and minister gathered for prayer and to say their final good-byes. Gary answered the door and was greeted by Louise asking for Albert's personal belongings. She had brought a list of things which she had given her son in years past which she now wanted to have returned.

Gary was stunned. Leaving the door open, he simply walked away, dumbfounded. The minister went to speak to Louise, unaware of what had just occurred. Louise explained to the minister the purpose of her visit. Explaining that Albert was near death, the minister suggested that she might want to visit with her son. He offered to ask Albert's friends to wait in the living room so she could have privacy in Albert's bedroom. He further suggested that if she would like, he could be with her while she saw her son. Louise paused, thanked the minister for his kindness and left.

Neither Louise nor her husband attended their son's funeral. Gary did receive a letter from Louise after the funeral requesting that he return the things she had given Albert. Deciding that it wasn't worth the fight, Gary packed the things Louise had requested and left them at his doorstep on the day Louise said she would visit. Gary, in turn, spent the day with friends. Having been given power of attorney by Albert and being executor of Albert's estate, Gary requested that his attorney write Louise asking that she not harass him further.

About six months later, Gary received a phone call from Louise. She asked if he would take her to Albert's grave as she did not know were her son had been buried. They arranged a time to do so. After visiting Albert's grave, Louise asked Gary to join her for coffee. She asked Gary many questions about Albert's illness and death. After about an hour, they parted with Louise asking if they could talk again in the future. Gary consented readily.

During this meeting, Gary learned that Louise had been seeing a minister for pastoral counseling since Albert's death. This minister had recently conducted a memorial service for Albert. It seemed to Gary that somehow this service gave Louise whatever ability it was to call him and attempt to resolve the issues of Albert's death.

As can be inferred through this story, the issues to be resolved are really no different than those addressed in the preceding chapter. The difference is simply *when* they are addressed. Yet, there is a great loss which results from not moving through these issues while the person with AIDS is living. Such delay becomes an additional dimension for pastoral care.

Pastoral care at the time of death is a delicate ministry to provide. As pastoral ministers, we not only face our own inadequacies in the face of death, but we share with others when they are perhaps most vulnerable.

In the case of AIDS, whether it is early in the course of the illness, during the long haul, at the time of death or through bereavement, pastoral care is indeed a ministry of reconciliation.

This reconciliation is primarily among the many different people who have become part of the greater family system, both biological and chosen. It includes reconciliation of ideas, values and life perspectives which are often complex and divergent.

Perhaps the greatest qualification for this ministry is a heart open to accept, respect, challenge and integrate these perspectives and those who hold them. This ministry of reconciliation is indeed the pastoral challenge of AIDS.